Baking Soda

Mind Blowing Baking Soda Uses to Improve Your Health, Beauty, Cleaning, and More!

Jonathan S. Hunt

Contents

Chapter 1. Baking Soda Basics.....9

Chapter 2. Using it for Various Beauty Problems.........................12

Chapter 3. Numerous Cleaning Solutions to Use..............................34

Chapter 4. Health Hacks to Help You Out.................................57

Chapter 5. Some Deodorizing Uses...............................78

Chapter 6. Hacks for Food, Plants & Gardening...................................100

Chapter 7. Just A Few More to Try...............................122

Chapter 8. Tips & Tricks to Make it Easier...144

© Copyright 2019 by Jonathan S. Hunt- All rights reserved.

This document is geared toward providing exact and reliable information in regard to the topic and issue covered. The publication is sold with the idea that the publisher is not required to render accounting, officially permitted, or otherwise, qualified services. If advice is necessary, legal or professional, a practiced individual in the profession should be ordered.

- From a Declaration of Principles which was accepted and approved equally by a Committee of the American Bar Association and a Committee of Publishers and Associations.

In no way is it legal to reproduce, duplicate, or transmit any part of this document in either electronic means or in printed format. Recording of this publication is strictly prohibited and any storage of this document is not allowed unless with written permission from the publisher. All rights reserved.

The information provided herein is stated to be truthful and consistent, in that any liability, in terms of inattention or otherwise, by any usage or abuse of any policies, processes, or directions contained within is the solitary and utter responsibility of the recipient reader. Under no circumstances will any legal responsibility or blame be held against the publisher for any reparation, damages, or monetary loss due to the information herein, either directly or indirectly.

Respective authors own all copyrights not held by the publisher.

The information herein is offered for informational purposes solely, and is universal as so. The presentation of the information is without contract or any type of guarantee assurance.

The trademarks that are used are without any consent, and the publication of the trademark is without permission or backing by the trademark owner. All trademarks and brands within this book are for clarifying purposes only and are the owned by the owners themselves, not affiliated with this document.

Chapter 1. Baking Soda Basics

The first thing you should know about baking soda is that it is different than baking powder. If you are using baking soda hacks, you won't be able to use baking powder instead. They cause batter to rise differently, and you'll find out that they have uses outside of cooking as well that are different.

Why Use It:

Baking soda is cheap. It all boils down to it being a cheap, easy and useful hack for anyone. Many people already know that it can be a household cleaner, but there are many more uses for baking soda. You can get it right at your grocery store, but makes sure that its real baking soda and not baking powder. You have to have the right substance if you want any of these hacks to work.

Buying in bulk will actually help you to cut down on your expenses even more, and usually you need very little else besides water, cotton balls, and occasionally a spray bottle for application. Baking soda might have plain packaging and a cheap price tags, but it's actually versatile around the house. Many people just let their box of baking soda collect dust and go unused in the pantry. Instead, break it out and use it for hygiene to garden hacks.

The Difference Between Baking Powder & Baking Soda:

Baking powder actually has cream of tartar in it. It also includes a drying agent which is usually a starch. Neither of these are actually in baking soda. If you're using baking soda in a recipe that requires baking powder, you'd need to use cream of tartar. Because of the cream of tartar and the starch included in baking powder, you can't use it in baking soda recipes, including in hacks.

Chapter 2. Using it for Various Beauty Problems

Baking soda can actually be used for beauty products as well, and it's an easy hack to use that will save you a lot of money. Everyone knows that beauty products are expensive from toner to acne cream. It can cost you a fortune, but when you have baking soda instead, you'll cut corners without looking like it, which will save you time and money.

Hack #1 Make Clarifying Shampoo

There are many benefits of a clarifying shampoo, and that's because it takes the buildup in our hair, including mousses, sprays, dirt, and just grease that will help you to get rid of it. If you have oily hair or greasy hair, then you'll find that a normal shampoo may just not work.

You need to have a clarifying shampoo that will remove everything from your hair while still conditioning it slightly. Usually, they're expensive, which is one of the only downsides of clarifying shampoos. However, with this baking soda hack, it's inexpensive and easy to make sure your hair is taken care of.

Ingredients:

1. Current Shampoo
2. 3 Tablespoons of Baking Soda
3. 3 Tablespoons of Water

Directions:

1. You'll mix the three tablespoons of water and baking soda together first.
2. Then add in a few drops of your current shampoo and use in your hair like you would regularly.
3. You can add condition afterwards, then you're set to go.

Hack #2 A Simple Hair Repair

You'll find that your hair is damaged, especially after chlorine. Chlorine can have your hair splitting, and it affect just about any hair. However, you're more at risk if you fine, previously damaged hair, dry hair, color treated hair or even chemically treated hair such as if you got a relaxer or a perm. However, baking soda can help with damaged hair as well.

Ingredients:

1. 1 Pint Water
2. ½ Tablespoon Baking Soda

Directions:

1. Mix the water and the baking soda together thoroughly, and once your hair is wet, apply it like you would regular shampoo.
2. Rinse and repeat once. Do this after each time you went into the pool to fight off discoloration or dullness.

Hack #3 Nail Shine

Many people have dull fingernails or toenails, but you can keep them healthy and clean with baking soda. This will help you to keep from having to use something that will cost you too much money, and all you need to add to the baking soda is a little water to make the right paste.

Ingredients:

1. 2 Teaspoons Baking Soda
2. Dash Water

Directions:

1. Put the baking soda into a bowl, and then add water, mixing it up until you get a paste.
2. If your paste is too watery, add more baking soda. If it's too thick, add a little more water.
3. Take a nail brush, and scrub it on any stains or discolorations on your nails. Even if you don't see either of these, scrub a coat onto your nails to give them that healthy glow. You can even use it to remove small bits of nail polish.
4. Rinse your hands off, and your nails are sure to look better.

Hack #4 Cleansing Scrub

Many people struggle to get soft and smooth skin, and you may already be paying a lot of money for an exfoliator, but it's unnecessary. You can simply use baking soda and water to apply to your face, and you'll have a facial scrub that works just as well as any expensive one you buy from the store. This is especially helpful if you have oily skin or have trouble with blackheads. You can use this anywhere on your body.

Ingredients:

1. 1 Tablespoon Baking Soda
2. Dash Water

Directions:

1. Make sure to add the baking soda into the bowl first, and then add just enough water to make it into a paste.
2. Apply it on your face in a thin coat, being careful that it doesn't touch your eyes or lips.
3. Massage it into your skin using a circular motion.
4. Rinse it away, and repeat once.

Hack #5 A Dry Shampoo

There are many reasons to love a dry shampoo, and you'll fall in love with a dry shampoo as soon as you use it. If you've already used a dry shampoo, you probably already know exactly how expensive it can be. One of the biggest reasons that you have to like dry shampoo is that you're pretty much ready to go in a blink of the eye, and you can completely skip the suds. It also helps with humidity, helps you to create waves in your hair, and it's great if you don't have time to hop in the shower.

Ingredients:

1. Baking Soda

Directions:

1. It's as simple as putting in baking soda on your scalp or on oily areas, and soon your hair will be looking as good as new. It's a great fix after a workouts, and it's easy to stash baking soda right in your gym bag.

Hack #6 Skin Cleanser

This is a cleanser that is great for your skin, but it's even better if you have sensitive sin. It helps to moisturize, has anti-aging properties, soothes skin, purges bacteria, draws out toxins and even gently exfoliates your skin. The best part is that it's easy to make.

Ingredients:

2. 1 Teaspoon Baking Soda
3. 1 Teaspoon Honey, raw
4. 3 Tablespoons Coconut Oil, Organic

Directions:

1. Make sure your coconut oil is in a bowl, and then add in your honey, making sure to stir it well.
2. Add the baking soda in next, stirring it together.
3. Once it's all together, put it in an airtight container and store it at room temperature.
4. Apply to your skin in small circles to exfoliate, and then rinse it with warm water.
5. Dab your skin dry with a wash cloth, but do not rub as it can be damaging to your freshly cleansed skin.

Hack #7 Teeth Whitener

Baking soda can even help you to whiten your teeth, and it's perfectly safe to use. You can whiten your teeth from your own home, and it'll help to make sure you don't spend more money on expensive solutions that won't work nearly as well. Just make sure to do it at least once a day and up to twice a day if you want to notice fast results.

Ingredients:

1. Hydrogen Peroxide
2. ½ Teaspoon Baking Soda
3. Water

Directions:

1. Start by diluting your hydrogen peroxide, and then put it into a bowl with your half a teaspoon of baking soda. Make sure that the hydrogen peroxide is properly diluted or it could actually harm your teeth.
2. Mix the ingredients together until it turns into a paste. It should fluff up, so don't worry because it's normal.
3. Use your toothbrush, and apply the paste, but try to avoid the gum areas for as much as you can.
4. You should brush for ten minutes, and then gargle with fresh water.
5. Make it a part of your daily routine.

Hack #8 Underarm Whitening

Everyone always feels like their underarms are dirty, and if you're worried about it, don't try a bleaching agent. Baking soda is a natural way to whiten your underarms, which is great after you've finished shaving.

Ingredients:

1. 2 Tablespoons Baking Soda
2. 4 Tablespoons Coconut Oil

Directions:

1. Just mi everything together, and use it to scrub under your arms.
2. Make sure to scrub using a circular motion, which will help to get rid of rough ad dead skin that collects there
3. You should leave it to sit for anywhere between five to ten minutes.
4. Rinse it off, and pat it dry. You'll have whiter and softer armpits afterwards.

Hack #9 Lighten Dark Spots

Dark spots can cause you to feel bad about yourself and feel like you're older than you are. However, scars and dark spots can be removed, even if they're from older acne. All you need to do is use baking soda, and this simple paste is easy to use.

Ingredients:

1. 3 Tablespoons Water
2. 1 Tablespoon Baking Soda

Directions:

1. Mix together until it forms a paste, and apply it to the dark spots. You need to leave the paste on overnight, and then you can rinse it with warm water.

2. Pat the area dry, and excess oil and dead skin will be removed as well.

Hack #10 An Acne Cure

If you have an issue with acne, try this baking soda and honey cure. It'll help to take acne away right away, and the honey is going to heal the skin that the acne has damaged. It'll leave your skin both clear and soft, so you'll find that it helps after just one application.

Ingredients:

1. 2 Teaspoons Honey

2. 2 Teaspoons Baking Soda

Directions:

1. Take a bowl and mix the baking soda and honey together thoroughly, and then apply it to the affected area. You can use it as an all over face mask if you avoid your eyes and lips.
2. Let it sit for ten to fifteen minutes before rinsing it off with lukewarm water. Pat the area dry. For severe acne, try this treatment two to three times daily, and you should notice improvement after one application.

Hack #11 Skin Brightening

If you think your skin looks dull, there is a solution for it. You don't have to deal with dull skin that makes you feel bad about yourself, and the solution is right in your kitchen. You'll find that you just need three simple ingredients to brighten your skin and your outlook.

Ingredients:

1. 1 Teaspoon Lemon Juice
2. 3 Teaspoons Baking Soda
3. 3 Teaspoons Water

Directions:

1. Make a paste by mixing all ingredients into a bowl together.
2. Apply it to your skin like you would a facemask, and leave it on for five to eight minutes.
3. Rinse with lukewarm water, and pat the area dry to keep from damaging your skin. You should notice results after one application, but multiple applications over a few days does best.

Chapter 3. Numerous Cleaning Solutions to Use

There are many different ways that you can use baking soda around your house to make sure that everything sparkles and looks like new. Many cleaning solutions are too expensive, and they can be harmful to you when you're using them. The fumes are harmful, but it's also harmful if you're getting it on your hands. It can damage your skin, causing rashes, callouses, and sometimes even burs. When you're using baking soda, there's no worry of that happening.

Cleaning Solution #1 Mopping Floors

There's no reason to buy expensive or harmful floor cleaners. If you have hard wood floors that need mopped to look like they're new again, then baking soda is your answer. Just take your normal cleaning tool, and you'll be able to get started immediately.

Ingredients:

1. A Bucket of Warm Water
2. ½ Cup Baking Soda

Directions:

1. Make sure to get a bucket of warm water, and then add in the half a cup of baking soda.
2. Make sure it's mixed thoroughly, and then you can use it to mop the floors like you would normally.
3. Rinse the floor clean.

Cleaning Solution #2 Furniture Cleaning

Your furniture can start to look dingy too, but you can give any furniture a face lift with baking soda. Just make sure that you're using it lightly, and you can clean it after somethings spilled on it, or you can make sure to use it every week on your furniture to keep it clean.

Ingredients:

1. ½ Cup Water
2. 2 Teaspoons Baking Soda

Directions:

1. Dampen the sponge in the water. Do not mix the baking soda and water together.
2. Apply the baking soda onto the surface of the damp sponge, and clean your furniture that way.
3. Wipe it clean with a dry and clean cloth.

Cleaning Solution #3 Silverware Polish

If you have real silverware, you know the pains of keeping it clean, but its well worth it. This is why you'll find that baking soda can help you to clean your silverware. It's simple and really only takes a few minutes.

Ingredients:

1. 3 Teaspoons Water
2. 1 Teaspoon Baking Soda

Directions:

1. Mix your water and baking soda together. No matter how much you make up, it needs to stay three parts water and one part baking soda.
2. Dip in a clean rag, and use the solution on your silverware to polish it.
3. Make sure to polish each piece carefully, and don't miss a spot.

4.

Cleaning Solution #4 Oven Cleaner

Cleaning your oven can become a pain, but you don't need to worry about it. You'll need a spray bottle, but with this baking soda hack it's sure to clean even the hardest baked on stains.

Ingredients:

1. 1 Cup Baking Soda
2. ½ Cup Water

Direction:

1. Sprinkle the baking soda on the bottom of the oven.
2. Put the water in the spray bottle, and spray it over the baking soda.
3. Let it sit overnight, and then scrub it away in the morning, wiping away any residue. Some people find that rinsing will work if it's too baked on.

Cleaning Solution #5 Refresh Your Rugs

You can freshen your rugs with baking soda as well, and it'll help to keep your house smelling clean and fresh. You just put it on before you vacuum, and you're ready to go. There is no reason that you should have to change your schedule, either. You'll be able to just add it into your routine.

Ingredients:

1. 1 Cup Baking Soda

Directions:

2. It's really that easy with one simple ingredient. Just take the baking soda and sprinkle it over the area.
3. Let it sit for fifteen to thirty minutes, and then vacuum. Your house will be smelling fresh in no time at all.

Cleaning Solution #6 Get Rid of Crayon

If you have children, you know the horrors of their adorable crayon drawings being all over your freshly painted walls. Baking soda can help you with that as well, helping to make sure that you have everything you need to get through and get your walls looking like new again.

Ingredients:

1. ¼ Cup Baking Soda

Directions:

1. Just take a clean sponge, and dip it into water. Make sure to squeeze it out so that it won't actually run down your walls.
2. Then, you can sprinkle baking soda on the sponge, and clean your walls like you normally would.

Cleaning Solution #7 Cleaning Containers

If you are using plastic containers to store your food, you probably have more than a few that are stained up. Instead, you'll be able to use baking soda so that you don't have to throw them away.

Ingredients:

1. 8 Tablespoons Baking Soda
2. 2 Tablespoons Water

Directions:

1. Mix your baking soda and water together, and put it over the stains in the plastic containers.
2. Let them sit overnight, and then you can clean them off as you normally would in the morning. You should notice the stains are gone. Repeat if the stains are too stubborn.

Cleaning Solution #8 Toilet Cleaner

If you're having stubborn stains that make your toilet look dirtier than it is, then you're going to need to make sure that you get rid of them. All you need is vinegar, baking soda, and time.

Ingredients:

1. 1 Cup Baking Soda
2. 3 Tablespoons Vinegar

Directions:

1. Pour in one cup of baking soda into the toilet.
2. Then, let it sit for thirty to forty-five minutes.
3. Afterwards, spray vinegar into the water and clean like you normally would.

Cleaning Solution #9 Keep Sponges Fresh

If you're using sponges on a regular basis, you need to keep them fresh. Fresh sponges work better, and baking soda will not only make them smell fresh but it'll help to make sure that all of the bacteria that could be harmful to you and your family isn't festering inside your cleaning tool.

Ingredients:

1. 1 Quart Water
2. 4 Tablespoons Baking Soda

Directions:

1. Make sure that your water is warm, and then add in your four tablespoons of baking soda.
2. Place the sponge in the water, and leave it for two to three hours or overnight.
3. Squeeze the sponge out and let it dry before using it next.

Cleaning Solution #10 Car Wash

If you don't want to pay for an expensive car wash or use expensive soap, baking soda can be your car wash solution. So long as your car has a proper was on it, it won't hurt the paint, and it'll have your car sparkling in no time.

Ingredients:

1. 1 Quart Water
2. ¼ Cup Baking Soda

Directions:

1. Just mix it together and take your rag to your car. If you have a pressure washer, you can use that.
2. Then, rinse your car, and it's good as new. It's really that easy.

Cleaning Solution #11 Grout Cleaner

Cleaning your grout can be hard, and as soon as it's dingy it makes the entire room look horrible and old. So, you'll find that with these two ingredients and some patience, your grout will look like it was just put in.

Ingredients:

1. 2 Tablespoons Bleach
2. 6 Tablespoons Baking Soda

Directions:

1. Mix together, and use the resulting paste to clean your grout. A rag just won't cut it, and you'll need to make sure that you have a proper scrub brush to help.

Cleaning Solution #12 Removing Sweat Stains

Sweat stains make your clothes look that much worse, and if it's on white, you really are in a tough position. Of course, there's no reason to toss that shirt any longer. You can just use this baking soda remedy to help remove those sweat stains from anything white.

Ingredients:

2. 1 Cup Vinegar
3. ½ Cup Baking Soda
4. 1 Tablespoon Salt
5. 1 Tablespoon Hydrogen Peroxide

Directions:

1. Mix everything together, and then place the shirt in the bowl of the solution.
2. Let it soak for twenty to thirty minutes.
3. Then, wash like you normally would, and you should notice that the sweat stain is gone.

Cleaning Solution #13 Burnt Pot Solution

Everyone who's ever had problems in the kitchen has burnt a pot or two, and sometimes they just refuse to come clean. It's no longer a problem if you burn a pot, besides a ruined meal or two. Just clean your pots with this baking soda solution, and the burnt stains will go away with ease.

Ingredients:

1. 4 Teaspoons Hydrogen Peroxide
2. 8 Teaspoons Baking Soda

Directions:

1. Just pour it over the burnt pot.
2. Let it sit overnight, and then just rinse and wash clean. There's absolutely no

scrubbing involved. If you need more solution, just up the amounts.

Chapter 4. Health Hacks to Help You Out

There are still many uses for baking soda, so don't put the box back in your cabinet just yet. You should never forget you have the versatile product, and when you're running low, remember to buy more so it's always stocked in your cabinet. Baking soda can benefit your health as well as your house, so keep it out for whenever you need it.

Remedy #1 A Blackhead Remedy

You don't have to deal with blackheads, just like you don't have to deal with acne. It's not as simple as a baking soda paste, but you'll still find everything you need in your kitchen cabinet. Never deal with blackheads. Instead, knock them out.

Ingredients:

1. 1 Teaspoon Baking Soda
2. ½ Teaspoon Lemon Juice
3. ½ Teaspoon Honey, Raw

Directions:

1. Sprinkle the baking soda into a bowl over the honey, and then add in the lemon juice.
2. Mix together, and apply it over the affected area.
3. Let it sit for five to ten minutes, and then you lightly wash it off with warm water, patting it dry.

Remedy #2 A Detox Bath

Everyone could use a detox bath now and again. Detox baths help to get rid of toxins in your body, and it helps you to feel better. It can decrease your stress levels, boost your immune system, and make you feel relaxed enough to get the sleep you need. It can even sooth your muscles.

Ingredients:

1. 1 Cup Baking Soda
2. 6-8 Drops Peppermint Essential Oil
3. 2 Cups Epsom Salts, Lavender Scented

Directions:

1. Draw your bath, and then put in your baking soda and Epsom salts first, making sure to mix them throughout the hot water.
2. Add in your essential oil, and soak for twenty to thirty minutes in the warm water before proceeding like normal.

Remedy #3 Treating Athlete's Foot

Athlete's foot is embarrassing, and it's very uncomfortable. It's best to catch athlete's foot and cure it before it gets too bad. Otherwise, it'll take more treatments to try and get rid of it.

This natural baking soda remedy is proven to work better than over the counter treatments, and it'll help you to alleviate and get rid of your athlete's foot fast.

Ingredients:

1. 5 Tablespoons Baking Soda
2. ¼ Cup Apple Cider Vinegar
3. 2 Cups Hot Water

Directions:

1. Prepare your water by adding in the apple cider vinegar and the baking soda, making sure it's mixed well.
2. Then, put your feet in the mixture, soaking for at least twenty minutes, making sure the affected area is submerged.
3. Pat the area dry, and do so two to three times daily.

Remedy #4 Removing Foot Odor

For those who deal with embarrassing foot odor, you've probably tried various remedies. However, this baking soda remedy is sure to work. Your foot odor will be gone after one application, and you can reapply it as much as necessary.

Ingredients:

1. ¼ Cup Baking Soda
2. 2 Teaspoons Rosemary
3. 8 Cups Water, Warm
4. 4 Tablespoons Lemon Juice, Fresh

Directions:

1. Add everything together, making sure that it's mixed thoroughly. If you want this soak to be more invigorating, you can always add a few drops of peppermint extract or essential oil.

2. Make sure to soak your feet for fifteen to twenty minutes, and then lightly scrub your feet. You should notice immediate relief from both itchiness and any previous odor.
3. Gently dry off your feet.

Remedy #5 Toenail Fungus Relief

Toenail fungus is more than just embarrassing. It's actually painful, and no one wants to deal with it any longer than they have to. If you're looking for quick and natural toenail fungus remedy, then baking soda is one of the main ingredients that you'll need. The remedy below is sure to help.

Ingredients:

1. 5 Tablespoons Baking Soda
2. 1 Cup White Vinegar
3. 2 Cups Water
4. 1 Teaspoon Tea Tree Oil

Directions:

1. Mix everything together, and make sure the water is warm. This will help you to both relax your feet and get rid of your toenail fungus.
2. Soak for twenty to thirty minutes, and then pat dry with paper towels.

Remedy #6 Getting Rid of Ringworm

Ringworm is painful, and it's very hard to actually get rid of. Many prescription and over the counter medications don't work, and those that do leave your skin, dry and irritated, as well as there being various side effects that you shouldn't have to deal with. With this baking soda remedy, you'll get rid of your ringworm quickly, and it'll help you to feel better quicker.

Ingredients:

1. 4 Tablespoons Baking Soda
2. 2 Tablespoons Hydrogen Peroxide

Directions:

1. Just put it all into a mixing bowl, and make sure to mix it all together until a thick paste is formed.
2. Put it over the affected area, and tape gauze to it, so that it's fully covered.
3. Leave it on, and replace it twice daily. Each time you replace it, wash it gently with warm water.

Remedy #7 Sore Feet Soak

If you have sore or aching feet, you don't have to deal with it. You can find a way to get rid of it quickly, and everything you need you probably already have in your kitchen. Soak your feet while you're reading, watching TV, or just relaxing with your family. It only takes twenty to thirty minutes, and your feet will feel better even after a long day.

Ingredients:

1. 3-4 Tablespoons Baking Soda
2. 1 Tablespoon Peppermint Essential Oil
3. 1 Tablespoon Sea Salt, Fine

4. 2 Cups Warm Water
5.

Directions:

1. Pour everything together, making sure to mix it well.
2. Soak your feet for at least twenty minutes, but soaking for thirty minutes will provide better results.

Remedy #8 Bee Sting Relief

Bee stings hurt, and there's no way to avoid them sometimes. However, there is a way to take the pain away almost immediately, and it doesn't require you to buy any costly items.

You'll have almost everything you need probably already in your pantry, so you can make the mixture up quick for quick relief. Meat tenderizer is added because it papain, which breaks down the toxin in bee stings, and the baking soda helps to draw it out.

Ingredients:

1. 1 Teaspoon Baking Soda
2. ½ Teaspoon Meat Tenderizer
3. 1 Teaspoon White Vinegar

Direction:

1. Mix everything together, and apply the resulting paste onto the affected area.
2. Next, make sure to place a sterile gauze pad over it and tape it down.
3. Remove after an hour or two, and the stinger will usually come right out as well if you have yet to remove it.

Remedy #9 Sunburn Relief Fast

Sunburn hurts, and you'll find that there are ways to help make sure that it goes away a little faster. Baking soda is known to help pull out the burning sensation, and it'll help you to feel better quick with as little damage to your skin as possible. You should notice immediate relief after the first application.

Ingredients:

1. 2 Teaspoons Baking Soda
2. ½ Teaspoon White Vinegar
3. 1 Teaspoon Water

Directions:

1. Mix everything together, and it should form a thick paste. Apply it to the affected area.
2. Let it dry for ten to fifteen minutes before gently removing it with cool water.

3. Apply three to four times daily until your sunburn is better.

Remedy #10 Ridding Yourself of a Sore Throat

You can get rid of a sore throat naturally and fast, and it's a cheap and easy solution. It only takes a few minutes, and you can add it into your routine throughout the day to provide needed relief and help you to even cure your sore throat by eliminating the acids that are causing you pain and killing off bacteria.

Ingredients:

1. 4 Ounces Warm Water
2. ½ Teaspoon Sea Salt, Fine
3. 1 Teaspoon Baking Soda

Directions:

1. Make sure to mix everting together, and then gargle.
2. Do not swallow, and do this two to three times daily for relief.

Remedy #11 Jellyfish Sting Remedy

A jellyfish sting hurts, and sometimes you don't want to use urine to get it to go away. So, baking soda can help you without needing embarrassing help. It's easy to use, and it's easy to make, so you'll get relief fast from even the worst sting in the worst area.

Ingredients:

1. 1 Teaspoon White Vinegar
2. 2 Teaspoons Baking Soda

Directions:

1. Mix together to make a paste, and then apply it to the area.
2. Let it sit for ten to fifteen minutes, and then wash with cool water, making sure to pat it dry. Reapply as necessary.

Chapter 5. Some Deodorizing Uses

Baking soda is great for deodorizing more than just your feet, and you'll find that there are many deodorizing baking soda uses. They can even be customized to fit your needs and personality. Essential oils are sometimes needed, but you'll find various deodorizing recipes in this chapter for anything from your carpet to your underarms, helping you to smell fresh personally as well as keep your home smelling clean all the time, even if you have pets.

Recipe #1 An Odor Absorber

If you have odors just floating around in your house due to kids, pets, or even just guests, you'll find that odor absorbers can be a life saver. It'll help you to remove odors from the air instead of just covering them up, which will make your house seem that much cleaner, and it'll make you more comfortable in your home.

Ingredients:

1. 1 Cup Baking Soda
2. 10 Drops Peppermint Essential Oil
3. 5-8 Drops Lemon Essential Oil
4. 6-8 Drops Orange Essential Oil

Directions:

1. Take a clean glass jar with a lid, and pour in your baking soda.
2. Add in all of your essential oils, making sure to mix together well.
3. Then, take the lid punching holes into it, and cover the mixture.
4. Sit it out, and you'll notice the odors disappearing.

Recipe #2 Carpet Deodorizer

This is a rose scented carpet deodorizer, but you can substitute your favorite essential oil if you don't want your house smelling like roses.

It's easy to make, and you can even make it up in advance, as it won't go bad.

Ingredients:

1. 2 Cups Baking Soda
2. 15-20 Drops Rose Essential Oil

Directions:

1. Just mix it all together, making sure that it doesn't clump.
2. The essential oil should be mixed throughout evenly, and you'll want to store it in an airtight container.
3. Sprinkle it over your carpet whenever it starts to smell bad. It can be before or after you vacuum, but make sure that it at least sits for twenty minutes before vacuuming. If you aren't going to vacuum afterwards, shake only a thin layer that will disappear into the carpet after walking over it.

Recipe #3 Fridge Deodorizer

Everyone who has ever had to deal with a fridge, especially with a large family, knows that sometimes it needs freshened up. This can happen even if you've cleaned it recently, so having a way to freshen up your fridge is always important and useful. Baking soda, once again, can easily do the trick.

Ingredients:

1. 10-20 Drops Lemon Essential Oil
2. 5-10 Drops Orange Essential Oil
3. ½ Cup Baking Soda

Directions:

1. Take an open container, and mix everything together. Try to keep the baking soda from clumping.
2. Place the open container with the mixture at the back of your fridge, and replace it every two weeks.

Recipe #4 Deodorize Your Shoes

You can use baking soda in a better way than just sprinkling it in the soles of your shoes. There is a less messy and quite effective way, and all you need is some coffee filters, string, and the ingredients below.

Ingredients:

1. 1 Cup Baking Soda
2. 10 Drops Jasmine Essential Oil
3. 5-6 Drops Rose Essential Oil

Directions:

1. Mix all of the essential oils into the baking soda, and then place it in three to four coffee filters.
2. Then, bag it up and tie a ribbon around it. Place it in your shoes. Each bag should last about two to four weeks.

Recipe #5 Mattress Freshener

If your mattress is starting to smell funky, then you need to find a way to freshen it that isn't going to actually hurt your mattress. This is a gentle freshener that is sure to eliminate any odor problems you may be dealing with. The best part is that you can use it as much as you want, including on your comforter, curtains, and even your pillows.

Ingredients:

1. 1 Tablespoon Baking Soda
2. 10-15 Drops Jasmine Essential Oil
3. 1 Tablespoon White Vinegar

4. 2 Cups Water, Distilled

Directions:

1. Mix everything together, and put it into a spray bottle.
2. Spray it on the area as needed. Remember that you can make this up in advance.

Recipe #6 Coconut Oil Deodorant

Coconut oil is meant to give your skin a soft and new look about it, and it can work in your baking soda deodorant as well. You'll be able to make it quickly, and with the right container take it with you, even to the gym. This baking soda recipe is easy to use, and it's even easier to make.

Ingredients:

1. ¼ Cup Baking Soda
2. 6 Tablespoons Coconut Oil
3. ¼ Cup Cornstarch
4. 6 Drops Jasmine Essential Oil

Directions:

1. Mix everything together, and if you need to heat up the coconut oil just slightly.
2. Store in an airtight container, and rub onto your armpits when necessary, as you normally would your deodorant.

Recipe #7 A Gentler Deodorant

Remember that if you're a girl, the lavender essential oil is sure to be a hit, but if you're a boy try using something like tea tree oil or sandalwood essential oil. This will give you a much more manly scent, but either way it's a great deodorant for sensitive skin.

Ingredients:

1. 1 Tablespoon Shea Butter
2. 1 Tablespoon Beeswax, Grated
3. 1 Tablespoon Coconut Oil, Extra Virgin
4. 2 Teaspoons Arrowroot Powder
5. 8-12 Drops Lavender Essential Oil

Directions:

1. Heat all of your liquid ingredients in a saucepan over low heat.
2. Add in your arrowroot powder, making sure to mix it all together.
3. Transfer to proper containers, and let cool before using.

Recipe #8 An Earthy Deodorant

You can smell earthy and good at the same time. There's no reason that you have to smell fruity or flowery, and this is a great, easy do it yourself baking soda deodorant recipe that you can use. It even works great as a gift.

Ingredients:

1. 5-8 Drops Rosemary Essential Oil
2. 10 Drops Sage Essential Oil
3. 2-4 Drops Lemongrass Essential Oil
4. 2 Tablespoons Coconut Oil
5. 1 Tablespoon Beeswax, Grated
6. 3 Teaspoons Baking Soda

Directions:

1. Heat all liquid ingredients together over low heat in a small saucepan.
2. Add in your beeswax, making sure to mix it throughout.
3. Add in the baking soda, mixing and then put it in the right containers, letting it cool before using it.

Recipe #9 Deodorize Your Cutting Board

Your cutting board is where you cut your meat, your vegetables, and even your fruit. It makes sense that odors will stick to it from raw meat, onions, or anything else being cut on it. So, you'll find that baking soda is able to be sued.

Ingredients:

1. Baking Soda
2. 1 Teaspoon Lemon Juice
3. 4 Ounces Water

Directions:

1. Take the baking soda and sprinkle it over your cutting board.
2. Take the lemon juice and add it into the water, putting it into a spray bottle.
3. Spray it over the baking soda, and let sit for about five minutes.
4. Wash and scrub it away like you normally would.

Recipe #10 Deodorize Your Vacuum Cleaner

Your vacuum cleaner is always collecting dirt and helping to clean your home, but because of it you'll find that it will often have an odor. It'll help your carpet a little as well, but you don't need to let it sit on your carpet or floors to help make sure it helps the vacuum.

Ingredients:

1. 2 Cups Baking Soda

Directions:

1. Sprinkle the baking soda where you're about to vacuum.
2. Then, pull out the vacuum and start to vacuum it up. this will help to get rid of any smells that your vacuum is holding, and you can do this anytime your vacuum needs to be freshened up a little bit.

Recipe #11 Deodorize Pet Bedding

Your pets like their smell, but that doesn't mean you have to. If you have a pet, then it's likely that their bedding is starting to cause an odor in your home. You can deodorize it safely for both you and your pet with baking soda, and this recipe will show you how.

Ingredients:

1. 1 Cup Baking Soda
2. ½ Teaspoon Lemon Juice

Directions:

1. Mix the baking soda and lemon juice together. Try to avoid clumping. Remember that you can use baking soda on its own.

2. Sprinkle it over the bedding, and then vacuum it up after waiting at least ten to fifteen minutes. It's safe for your pets to use immediately.

Recipe #12 A Closet Freshener

This isn't just a closet freshener, but it'll actually help to ward off moths because of the particular essential oil that you're using as well. Lavender helps to ward off moths, and it'll keep your clothes fresh and moth free. You won't have to worry about any musky smell anymore.

Ingredients:

1. 15-20 Drops Lavender Essential Oil
2. 1 Cup Baking Powder

Directions:

1. Mix in the lavender oil to the baking soda, and try to break up any clumps.
2. Next, place it in an open container, putting it into your closet. Make sure you put it somewhere where you won't knock it over.

Chapter 6. Hacks for Food, Plants & Gardening

There are still gardening, food, and plant tips that you can use when dealing with baking soda. Baking soda is versatile for inside and outside your house. It can help you with dealing with ants, keeping roses fresh, and making sure that your meat is tender. It's truly versatile, and often, it's simple to use.

Hack #1 Sweeten Your Tomatoes

If you are trying to grow tomatoes, it can be hard to make them sweet, but a little bit of baking soda will go a long ways with this hack. The reasons that tomatoes usually turn out bitter is because of the high acidity level, but baking soda can help to make sure that the acidity is lowered.

Ingredients:

1. ¼ Cup Baking Soda

Directions:

1. Make sure to sprinkle some of the baking soda lightly in the soil and turn it where your tomatoes are.
2. Do not sprinkle too much, or it can hurt your tomatoes instead of help them. Do so every few weeks, or after it rains to make sure it's not washed away.

Hack #2 Keep Slugs Away

Slugs can harm your plants, and no one likes to deal with them in your garden. Of course, you'll find that baking soda can help with this as well. It's easy to keep slugs away from your plants, so you don't have to worry about them getting eaten up anymore.

Ingredients:

1. Baking Soda

Directions:

1. Every time you see a slug, all you have to do is pour baking soda on them. If you have an infestation, this is a great way to get rid of them quickly. Some people believe that it will help if you make a line around your plants, but it's proven to be more effective it's applied directly to the slug.

Hack #3 An Organic Pesticide

If you're looking for a safe and organic pesticide to help you with your garden, then you'll find that baking soda is one of the main ingredients. It's a two ingredient pesticide that can be made in advance, and it's extremely simple to use and make. Just make sure that you have a spray bottle on hand. You can use any cooking oil, but vegetable oil is easy to get ahold of and relatively cheap.

Ingredients:

1. 1 Teaspoon Baking Soda
2. 1/3 Cup Vegetable Oil

Directions:

1. Make the mixture up in advance, and label it.
2. Then, take two teaspoons of the mixture, mixing it to a cup of water.
3. Spray over your plants every week. Some people use it every four to five days, and it'll keep pests away.

Hack #4 Keep Roses Healthy

You'll find that your roses, when you're growing them, can have a powdery mildew. You may even get them from the store that way, and this spray will help with that as well. It's a simple spray that you can use on growing roses to help them stay healthy and keep this mildew away.

Ingredients:

1. 7 Tablespoons Baking Soda
2. 5 Gallons Water
3. 2 Teaspoons Vegetable Oil

Directions:

1. Make sure to mix everything together, and mix it thoroughly.

2. Spray it on your roses every week using a spray bottle.
3. Look out for any signs of burning on your roses. You can use it once weekly if there is no burning. If burning occurs, you need to space it out.

Hack #5 Battling Compost Smell

If you're using a compost to help your garden, then you're going to want to find a way that will help you to keep the smell down. Compost is great for your soil, but it's not so good for your nose. This wonderful solution is easy, and you won't have to worry about your yard smelling like it would without it.

Ingredients:

1. Baking Soda

Directions:

1. Adding baking soda to your compost is good for soil, and if you want to keep the smelly odor down, just add the baking soda into it and mix it. Just sprinkle it on right out of the box.

Hack #6 Clean Clay Pots

If you have clay pots or bird baths because of a nice garden, you're going to want to keep them nice by keeping them clean. If you're cleaning something birds use or you need cleaned for a plant, it's best you don't use toxic chemicals. That's why baking soda comes in handy.

Ingredients:

1. 5 Tablespoons Baking Soda
2. ½ Cup Water

Directions:

1. Mix it together, and use a scrub brush and solution on the clay pots and even a bird bath. You ca also use a damp cloth if it's delicate.

Hack #7 Keep Soil Fresh

If you love to garden, then you now that it's important that the soil stays fresh. Fresh soil helps to keep your plants healthy, and if you're using it for any crop, it's even more important.

Ingredients:

1. 1 Tablespoon Baking Soda

Directions:

1. Just sprinkle the baking soda on the clay pot before you put the soil in it. It should be a thin layer. You may have to use more or less baking soda depending on the size of the pot you're using. This will help your plants to grow a little better.

Hack #8 For Ants

Everyone has a problem with ants here or there, but there's no reason to buy expensive and harmful chemicals. Baking soda is a great way to battle ants without any harmful chemicals in your home or around your plants.

Ingredients:

1. 1 Cup Baking Soda
2. 1 Teaspoon Vinegar

Directions:

1. Add baking soda to the ant hill when it's damp.
2. Then, pour on the vinegar. If you need to, you can make the ant hill damp.

Hack #9 Homemade Scouring Powder

There are many reasons that you may want scouring powder, as there are many ways it can be used in your home. Many bought scouring powders are too rough, but this is a slightly gentler one that you can easily make at home. Baking soda is just one of the three ingredients that you'll need.

Ingredients:

1. 1 Cup Borax
2. 1 Cup Sea Salt, Fine
3. 1 Cup Baking Powder

Directions:

1. Mix together, and then put it in an airtight container, storing it until it's needed.

Hack #10 Clean Your BBQ Grill

IF you're looking for a way to easily and cheaply clean your BBQ grill, you'll find that baking soda once again has a miracle solution that you can use It helps to clean the grease off, and all you need is a wire brush.

Ingredients:

1. 4 Tablespoons Water
2. 8 Tablespoons Baking Soda

Directions:

1. Mix it together to make a paste, and then you can take a wire brush and clean your grill with it.
2. Let it sit for ten to fifteen minutes before wiping it away.
3. Before cooking food on the grill again, turn it on for a moment to help get rid of any leftover residue of the paste before cooking.

Hack #11 Peeling Eggs Made Easy

If you like hard boiled eggs, it doesn't mean that you have to like peeling them. Peeling hard boiled eggs can become more of a hassle, and they don't usually turn out looking pretty, which can affect some recipes. However, once again baking soda can come to your rescue.

Ingredients:

1. 1 Teaspoon Baking Soda

Directions:

1. A teaspoon of baking soda is all you need, and you'll want to put it in the water when you're cooking your boiled eggs.

2. Ice the boiled eggs when you're done, and then peel. You should notice that the shells come off much easier.

Hack #12 Neutralizing Beans

You may like beans without beans liking you. All you have to do is add it to the soak when you're using dried beans, and you'll notice less gas and bloating when you cook and eat them. Baking soda, once again, comes to the rescue.

Ingredients:

1. ½ Teaspoon Baking Soda

Directions:

1. Just add the half a teaspoon of baking soda to your overnight soak when you put your dried beans into it.
2. Continue with the soak and cooking like you normally would.

Hack #13 Vegetable & Fruit Wash

You should always wash your vegetables and fruits before you use them, but you need a wash that is gentle. Once again, baking soda can come to your rescue. It's better than just rinsing, and it'll make sure you aren't ingesting any harmful pesticides when you cook or just eat these vegetables and fruit.

Ingredients:

1. 3 Cups Cool Water
2. 2 Tablespoons Baking Soda

Directions:

1. Take a clean bowl, and then put the cool water in it, mixing in the baking soda.
2. Place any fruits or vegetables you need washed inside it, and let them sit for ten to twenty minutes.

3. Pat the fruits and vegetables dry before putting them away. This will help to remove pests and chemicals.

Chapter 7. Just A Few More to Try

There are still many useful things that baking soda can do for you, and you'll find a few more helpful hacks to try in this chapter. It'll help you with various things in and outside your house, and by now you're probably realizing just how versatile baking soda really is. Being cheap and versatile makes it a must for your home.

Hack #1 Fluff Your Omelets

If you love eating omelets, then you're going to want to make them fluffy. It's going to give you an edge when you show off to your friends or loved ones, and it'll help you to look a little more competent in the kitchen.

Ingredients:

1. 3 Eggs
2. ½ Teaspoon Baking Soda

Directions:

1. Cook your omelets like you normally would, and when you do, just make sure

to add a half a teaspoon to every three eggs. Do not add more, as it will then change the taste of your food.

Hack #2 Remove the Taste of Wild Game

If you love to hunt, it doesn't mean that you have to love the gamey smell. You can remove it, and a baking soda solution is yet another miracle solution for this issue. So, make sure to try it the next time you have fresh caught rabbit or deer.

Ingredients:

1. 1 Teaspoon
2. 1 Cup Water

Directions:

1. Mix it together and making a baking soda solution that you can soak your wild game in.
2. Make sure to soak for at least five to six hours, but you can soak overnight, and it will help to tenderize your meat as well.

Hack #3 Homemade Toothpaste

If you're looking for a homemade toothpaste, then you'll find that baking soda can do the trick. At the same time, it'll help you to make sure that you're whitening your teeth while keeping them clean. The peppermint extract will help to remove the baking soda taste.

Ingredients:

1. 1 Teaspoon Baking Soda
2. ½ Teaspoon Water
3. ¼ Teaspoon Peppermint Extract

Directions:

1. Mix it all together as you make a paste out of the ingredients.
2. Dip your toothbrush into the newly made paste, and brush your teeth like you normally would.

Hack #4 Relieve Itching

It doesn't usually matter why you're itching because you shouldn't have to deal with it. Baking soda will relieve itching fast, and it'll help you to get the relief you need to go about your day. It's as simple as making a simple paste.

Ingredients:

1. 1 Teaspoon Baking Soda
2. 1 Teaspoon Water

Directions:

1. Take a clean bowl, and mix it into a paste, making sure that it's thick. Add more baking soda if necessary and continue to mix until you get the proper consistency.
2. Apply the paste onto the area of your skin that's itching.
3. Let it sit for five to ten minutes.

4. Gently wash it off with lukewarm water, and pat the area dry with paper towels.

Hack #5 Freshen Your Breath

If you don't want to deal with bad breath, you simply don't have to. You don't need peppermint mouthwash to get the right smelling breath, and a baking soda solution really does do the trick.

Ingredients:

1. ½ Teaspoon Baking Soda
2. 4 Ounces Water

Directions:

1. Mix it together, and then gargle with the solution. Do this twice, and just add it into your normal routine.

Hack #6 Deodorize & Prevent Smoldering

If you smoke, then you have to worry about smoldering in your ashtray as well as deodorizing. Baking soda can once again come to your rescue, and it's easy to use to make sure that your house doesn't start to smell like smoke.

Ingredients:

1. 1 Teaspoon Baking Soda

Directions:

1. To make sure to get rid of the odor and prevent smoldering, every once in a

while make sure to sprinkle a little bit of baking soda in your ashtray. It'll also help to keep the smell of smoke from infesting your house.

Hack #7 Repel Cockroaches

You shouldn't have to deal with cockroaches anymore, and you don't if you have a bit of baking soda. Just make sure that you sprinkle it where you need to, and it's extremely easy to use. Just remember to act quickly because if you don't, cockroaches easily turn into an infestation that gets into every room of your house, and they're much harder to get rid of when it progresses this far.

Ingredients:

1. 2 Tablespoons Baking Soda

Directions:

1. Every time you feel that cockroaches are somewhere, you need to sprinkle baking soda in the area.
2. You'll want to put it under sinks and in kitchen cabinets even if you can't see where they're coming from, as these are likely places for cockroaches to be hiding.

Hack #8 Rabbit Repellent

If you are trying to grow a lush and fruitful garden, then you can't afford for anything to be eating your vegetables and fruits, including cute rabbits. You can repel them by using baking soda as well. It's really as easy as having that one little box ready to use in your cabinet.

Ingredients:

1. 1 Cup Baking Soda

Directions:

1. Remember that rabbits will eat almost anything, so sprinkle it around your plants so that they don't try to eat your fruits and vegetables. You'll have to replace it after it rains, and you'll need to do so at least once every other week.

Hack #9 Save Old Books

If you love to read, you probably have more than a few old books in your collection. Sadly, you probably know how easy it is for mold to grow in the pages causing you to need to throw them out. Baking soda can rescue these books, and it's a simple and easy solution to use. Save your books with this baking soda hack.

Ingredients:

1. 2 Cups Baking Soda

Directions:

1. Seal your books in an airtight container, making sure the baking soda is spread evenly at the bottom. This will save your books from molding as well as get rid of the odor that many old books have.

Hack #10 Quick Dog Bath

Just like how baking soda helps to make sure that you have a dry shampoo, it can work for your dog as well. You can't always give your dog a bag, so using this recipe will make sure they don't smell.

Ingredients:

1. ¼ Cup Baking Soda

Directions:

2. Sprinkle your dog's coat lightly with baking soda, making sure to avoid their eyes and mouth.
3. Leave it for five minutes, and then take a brush and brush it out.

Hack #11 Melt Even Stubborn Ice

If you live somewhere where your driveway is icing frequently, you may not want to spend the money on something that will hardly work to de-ice it. However, baking soda can be your miracle cure once more, and it's cheaper than other alternatives as well.

Ingredients:

1. 6 Cups Baking Soda
2. 4 Cups Sand

Directions:

1. Just sprinkle baking soda onto the ice, and then put sand down for traction. This way there is no harmful chemicals to your plants, family, or even your pets.

Hack #12 Remove All Wine Stains

If you're a wine lover, then you have probably spilled wine a time or two, but you don't have to worry about it. Baking soda can get rid of even the most stubborn wine stain, and you won't have to worry about expensive chemicals or replacing the item. It even works on grease stains.

Ingredients:

1. 1 Cup Baking Soda
2. 2 Teaspoons Baking Soda
3. 1 Teaspoon Water

Directions:

1. Start by sprinkling your larger amount of baking soda onto the stain, and let it sit for about five to ten minutes.
2. Brush the baking soda away, and then make a paste using the water and baking soda.
3. Scrub the area with the paste, letting it sit for another ten minutes.
4. Continue to clean like you normally would.

Hack #13 Unclog Your Drains

Don't spend your money on chemicals that will harm your plumbing, and instead let baking soda be your remedy as well. You will have an unclogged sink in no time, and it's easy to do.

Ingredients:

1. 3 Cups Hot Water
2. ½ Cup Baking Soda
3. 1 Cup Hot Water
4. 1 Cup White Vinegar
5. 3 Cups Hot Water

Directions:

1. Start with your hot, nearly boiling water, and run it down your clogged drain.
2. Make a mixture of your half a cup of baking soda and one more cup hot water, and pour it down the drain. Bubbling is normal.
3. Boil three more cups of hot water, and pour it down your drain.

Chapter 8. Tips & Tricks to Make it Easier

Now you know various baking soda hacks that will make it easier for you to do things inside and outside the house, including treating ailments and boosting your hygiene. Baking soda is already an easy remedy to use, but there are a few things that you can do to make it even easier to use these hacks.

Buy in Bulk:

Everyone knows that baking soda is rather cheap, but if you're using it for too many things in your home, it's sure to go quickly. This is why you might want to consider buying in bulk if you see baking soda on sale. You can get baking soda at your local grocery store, but you can buy it online as well. Buying in bulk will save you money, and it'll help you to be able to use baking soda more often for everything that it has to offer you.

Label Different Boxes:

If you're using baking soda for everything, you may want a box for different things. For example, when you're using baking soda outdoors, you may want to keep it outdoors instead of inside. You won't want to use the same baking soda box that you put next to your compost heap in your kitchen to be used for baking. So make sure to label each box carefully if you're using it for a variety of things.

Keep Vinegar Around:

Many baking soda recipes that help you around the house require vinegar. You're going to want to keep it around so that you don't have to run to the store every time you want to use these recipes. So make sure that you have both white vinegar and apple cider vinegar with you. White vinegar is used more often, but there are some recipes that will only work if you have apple cider vinegar, and both of these products can also be bought in bulk if you're using them enough.

The Right Containers:

Having the right containers also will help to make sure that you have what you need to use any baking soda hacks right away. It's best to have airtight containers, such as glass mason jars, but smaller containers so long as they are tin and not plastic, will work as well. You may also want to have containers that have a top that will help you to sprinkle deodorizing mixtures as well as spray bottles for liquid baking soda hacks to help you in and outside the house.

Use baking soda hacks whenever you're having issues, and make sure to keep enough on hand.

Remember that any little store, grocery store, or even dollar store will usually have baking soda, but your best deals are usually at the supermarket. You probably already have a baking soda box sitting unused in your cabinet, so break it out and make your home and health a little better.

www.ingramcontent.com/pod-product-compliance
Lightning Source LLC
Chambersburg PA
CBHW052144110526
44591CB00012B/1855